Diagnosis of the Bleeding Patient:
Fast Focus Study Guide

JT Thomas, MD

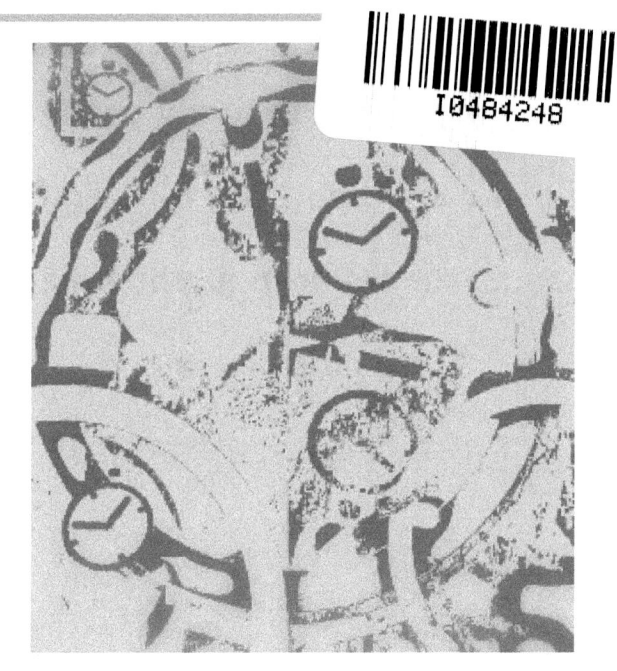

Acknowledgements

I dedicate this book to my beautiful wife and children, who I love more than all the water in all the oceans and all the seas.

CONTENTS

- This book is written to help the reader further understand the Diagnosis of the Bleeding Patient.

- This book is written in a simple and easy to read format designed for medical students, residents and physicians who are preparing for boards.

- This book simplifies a complicated medical issue so you will remember the important details.

- You will not get caught up in the minutia. Just the facts are found in this book.

- This Fast Focus Study Guide will provide you with a practical review of the key information you need to know.

- Buy this book now if you want this quick and concise information

When asked to see a bleeding patient there are several findings that are important to making the proper diagnosis.

Where is the patient bleeding (mucocutaneous, deep)?

What is the clinical scenario (recent surgery, sepsis, cancer)?

What has been done already in an attempt to stop the bleeding?

Has this ever happened to this patient before?

When thinking about these patients there are several questions that immediately come to mind that help narrow the differential diagnosis. In a surgical patient, is the bleeding a surgical complication or is something else responsible? Is the patient only bleeding at the site of the operation? Is there a disorder involving vascular integrity? Are there quantitative or qualitative platelet issues? Is the bleeding caused by a disorder of pro-coagulant factors or possibly a defects of fibrinolytic pathway?

Disorders of platelet number or function typically present with superficial bruising and mucocutaneous bleeding. The bleeding in these patients often occurs immediately after trauma. In patients with disorders of the coagulation proteins, there is typically deep tissue bleeding characterized by hematomas or hemarthrosis. This bleeding is often delayed.

Petechia are typically seen in patients with qualitative or quantitative platelet problems. In this setting the petechia do not blanch and are not raised. These petechia must be examined closely for signs of vasculitis where the lesions would actually be raised and palpable.

The abnormalities of hemostasis can be divided into disorders of vessel wall integrity, thrombocytopenia, platelet dysfunction, coagulopathy, and dysfunctional fibrinolysis.

Stages of Hemostasis

Vessel Wall Integrity

Adequate Numbers of Platelets

Proper Functioning Platelets

Adequate Levels of Clotting Factors

Proper Function of Fibrinolytic Pathway

Anticoagulation Effect

Vessel Wall Integrity

Vessel wall integrity can be disrupted in multiple situations. When the vessel wall does not function properly, blood cells extravasate into the subcutaneous tissue and the skin. Patients typically present with symptoms of petechial, purpura, and ecchymoses.

Vessel Wall Integrity

Cholesterol crystals can cause vessel wall injury secondary to cholesterol embolization resulting in symptoms including purpura, acral petechiae, peripheral ulcers, and livedo reticularis.

Vessel Wall Integrity

Disseminated intravascular coagulation (DIC) can cause vessel wall injury via both thrombotic and hemorrhagic mechanisms. Symptoms could include petechia, purpura, and ecchymosis, and hemorrhage.

Vessel Wall Integrity

Medications can be associated with allergic hypersensitivity resulting in blood vessel injury with petechiae and purpura.

Vessel Wall Integrity

Henoch Schonlein purpura is a leukocytoclastic vasculitis that causes vessel wall injury resulting in palpable purpura and hematuria, hemorrhagic vesicles or bullae.

Vessel Wall Integrity

Hypersensitivity vasculitis can cause palpable
purpura.

Vessel Wall Integrity

Bacterial, fungal, viral, rickettsial, protozoal, and parasitic infections can produce purpura with direct vascular invasion by the organism, disseminated intravascular coagulation, purpura fulminans, and immune complex vasculitis. Other mechanisms include septic emboli, direct effects of toxins released by the infecting organisms on the vasculature, and thrombocytopenia.

Vessel Wall Integrity

Amyloidosis is associated with light-chain (AL) deposits blood vessel wall infiltration with increased vascular fragility resulting in petechia and hemorrhagic lesions.

Vessel Wall Integrity

Ehler-Danlos syndrome is a connective tissue disorder associated with bruising.

Vessel Wall Integrity

Vitamin C deficiency is associated with defective collagen and ground substance formation resulting in petechia, and perifollicular purpura, ecchymoses, and mucous membrane purpura and hemorrhagic gingivitis.

Vessel Wall Integrity

Cushing syndrome and exogenous glucocorticoids can be associated with derma thinning and purpura.

Vessel Wall Integrity

Drug induced leukocytoclastic vasculitis has been associated with multiple medications.

Vessel Wall Integrity

Paraneoplastic vasculitis is characterized by a syndrome of petechiae, palpable purpura, urticaria, maculopapular lesions, leg ulcers, and/or erythema multiforme seen in association with cancer.

Vessel Wall Integrity

Chronic solar damage results in actinic purpura associated with decreased collagen, elastin, and ground substance due to aging.

Vessel Wall Integrity

The immune complexes of cryoglobulinemia may initiate alterations in endothelial cells resulting in increased vascular permeability, neutrophil infiltration, and vessel wall damage. This is associated with purpura, acral hemorrhagic necrosis, macular and palpable purpura, livedo reticularis, subungual hemorrhage, and hemorrhagic bullae.

Vessel Wall Integrity

Hereditary hemorrhagic telangiectasia is characterized by widespread dermal, mucosal, and visceral telangiectasias secondary to abnormalities in the endothelial protein endoglin. Gastrointestinal, oral, and urogenital bleeding occurs.

<u>Stages of Hemostasis</u>

Vessel Wall Integrity

Adequate Numbers of Platelets

Proper Functioning Platelets

Adequate Levels of Clotting Factors

Proper Function of Fibrinolytic Pathway

Anticoagulation Effect

Adequate Numbers of Platelets

Pseudothrombocytopenia caused by EDTA-dependent platelet agglutinins. Pseudothrombocytopenia is a common condition that must be excluded whenever a patient presents with low platelets. If needed the blood can be collected in a blue top tube that contains heparin rather than the purple tube that contains EDTA. You must remember that the dilution of blood collected in a blue top tube is different than the EDTA tube and the results will give results that are falsely low.

Adequate Numbers of Platelets

Thrombocytopenia occurs due to splenic pooling or sequestration. The thrombocytopenia associated with splenomegaly results from the displacement of a peripherally circulating platelets into a slowly exchangeable splenic pool.

Adequate Numbers of Platelets

Thrombocytopenia can occur in people receiving large volume red blood cell transfusion. The severity of thrombocytopenia is related to the number of red cell transfusions but is not simply a function of the dilution factor of massive transfusion.

Adequate Numbers of Platelets

Fanconi anemia is characterized by severe aplastic anemia with hypoplastic thrombocytopenia or pancytopenia. Patients with Fanconi anemia are at increased risk of developing leukemia and other malignancies. The disease generally results in death unless corrected by allogeneic marrow transplantation.

Adequate Numbers of Platelets

The May-Hegglin anomaly is characterized by giant platelets and characteristic leukocyte inclusion bodies often associated with thrombocytopenia.

Adequate Numbers of Platelets

Wiskott-Aldrich syndrome is an X-linked immunodeficiency syndrome characterized by thrombocytopenia, eczema, and immunodeficiency. These patients often have thrombocytopenia with small platelets.

Adequate Numbers of Platelets

Thrombocytopenia is common in patients with HIV infection characterized by ineffective platelet production caused by HIV infection of the auxiliary marrow cells resulting in diminished hematopoietic support by the marrow stroma.

Adequate Numbers of Platelets

Nutritional deficiency can result in thrombocytopenia. This occurs due to megaloblastic anemia related to vitamin B12 deficiency and alcohol related folic acid deficiency.

Adequate Numbers of Platelets

Thrombocytopenia in alcoholic patients is almost always due to cirrhosis with congestive splenomegaly or to folic acid deficiency. Some patients with thrombocytopenia may occur in the absence of nutritional deficiency or splenomegaly thought related to direct marrow suppression of platelet production..

Adequate Numbers of Platelets

Thrombotic thrombocytopenic purpura (TTP) is characterized by thrombotic microangiopathies with thrombocytopenia associated with microangiopathic hemolytic anemia. In the absence of ADAMTS13 there is increased concentration of long sticky VWF multimers accumulate and attach to platelets and causing formation of platelet thrombi that results in thrombocytopenia associated with microangiopathic hemolytic anemia.

Adequate Numbers of Platelets

Hemolytic uremic syndrome (HUS) presents with a triad of microangiopathic hemolytic anemia, thrombocytopenia and acute renal failure. Classic HUS is caused by Shiga toxin producing E coli. HUS typically presents with diarrhea with or without vomiting, irritability, bloody diarrhea, oliguria and hematuria. Atypical HUS is caused by dysregulation of the complement system associated with gain- or loss-of-function mutations of the alternative pathway.

Adequate Numbers of Platelets

Gestational Thrombocytopenia is characterized by thrombocytopenia: The presence of mild (Platelets usually >70k) and asymptomatic thrombocytopenia occurrence during late gestation with spontaneous resolution after delivery. This is generally considered a benign process during pregnancy and no specific intervention other than active surveillance during pregnancy is indicated.

Adequate Numbers of Platelets

Immune thrombocytopenia (ITP) is a condition that is characterized by antibody-mediated destruction of platelets associated with impaired megakaryocyte platelet production. IgG antiplatelet antibodies cause splenic sequestration and isolated thrombocytopenia.

Adequate Numbers of Platelets

Cyclic thrombocytopenias could possibly be an unusual manifestation of idiopathic (autoimmune) thrombocytopenic purpura. This disorder is most commonly seen in young women and is characterized by platelet decreased survival. This is typically a chronic condition.

Adequate Numbers of Platelets

Heparin induced thrombocytopenia is characterized by IgG antibodies against macromolecular complexes of platelet factor 4 (PF4) and heparin (H–PF4).

Adequate Numbers of Platelets

Drug induced thrombocytopenia is most commonly associated with an IgG antibody that occurs in response to an drug or the drug-platelet complex. This results in a rapid fall of platelet and sometimes this is associated with bleeding.

Stages of Hemostasis

Vessel Wall Integrity

Adequate Numbers of Platelets

Proper Functioning Platelets

Adequate Levels of Clotting Factors

Proper Function of Fibrinolytic Pathway

Anticoagulation Effect

Proper Functioning Platelets

Aspirin will irreversibly bind and inhibits the platelet cyclooxygenase (COX-1) enzyme. This results in diminished thromboxane A2 production and decreased platelet aggregation.

Proper Functioning Platelets

Von Willebrand disease is characterized by diminished or dysfunctional von Willebrand protein. This protein normally functions to mediate the adhesion of platelets to collagen exposed on the endothelial cell surface. In addition, von Willebrand protein binds to and stabilizes factor VIII in circulation.

Proper Functioning Platelets

Glanzmann thrombasthenia is characterized by a defect in the platelet GPIIb-GPIIIa complex that results from failure of platelets to bind fibrinogen and aggregate with physiological agonist such as ADP, thrombin, epinephrine or collagen. There is aggregation with ristocetin. The disorder is inherited in an autosomal recessive manner. Treatment of the disorder includes the application of pressure to the site of bleeding. Platelet transfusion may be useful in some circumstances.

Proper Functioning Platelets

Bernard-Soulier is a giant platelet syndrome characterized by either a decrease or absence of all four proteins of the platelet surface glycoprotein complex identified as the GPIb complex that acts as a binding site for von Willebrand factor. This is inherited in an autosomal recessive manner. Platelet aggregation studies show normal aggregation in the setting of ADP, and collagen. The platelets do not aggregate proplely with risotectin. Treatment of bleeding in Bernard-Soulier patients is improved with application of pressure, topical thrombin and platelet transfusion.

Stages of Hemostasis

Vessel Wall Integrity

Adequate Numbers of Platelets

Proper Functioning Platelets

Adequate Levels of Clotting Factors

Proper Function of Fibrinolytic Pathway

Anticoagulation Effect

Adequate Levels of Clotting Factors

The PT and PTT are used to screen for adequate levels of clotting factors. The results of an abnormal PT or PTT should always be verified using a mixing study.

Adequate Levels of Clotting Factors

A patient with an abnormal PT and a normal PTT should undergo a mixing study. If the mixing study is normal, then test factor VII activity.

Adequate Levels of Clotting Factors

A patient with an normal PT and a prolonged PTT should undergo a mixing study. If the mixing study is normal then test for factor VIII, factor IX, and factor XI activity.

Adequate Levels of Clotting Factors

A patient with an abnormal PT and an abnormal PTT should undergo a mixing study. If the mixing study is normal then Test factor V, factor X, and factor II (prothrombin) activity.

Adequate Levels of Clotting Factors

If the patient has symptoms that are concerning for abnormal levels of clotting factors, but the PT and PTT are normal, then test factor XIII activity and consider checking the clot solubility assay.

Adequate Levels of Clotting Factors

The prothrombin time (PT) is evaluates the extrinsic pathway and the common pathway.

Adequate Levels of Clotting Factors

The activated partial thromboplastin (PTT) evaluates the intrinsic pathway and the common pathway.

Adequate Levels of Clotting Factors

The thrombin time (TT) measures the final step of the clotting pathway, the conversion of fibrinogen to fibrin. A prolonged thrombin time can be caused by anticoagulants, the presence of fibrin/fibrinogen degredation products, Hypofibrinogenemia (<100 mg/dL), dysfibrinogenemia, or hyperfibrinogenemia (>400 mg/dL), elevated concentrations of serum proteins, as occurs in multiple myeloma or amyloidosis, thrombin antibodies.

Adequate Levels of Clotting Factors

Reptilase time (RT) is similar to the thrombin time in measuring the conversion of fibrinogen to fibrin. The reptilase time is useful for detecting abnormalities in fibrinogen and in detecting the presence of heparin (heparin will cause prolongation of the TT but not RT). The reptilase time is most useful for determining if heparin is the cause of a prolonged thrombin time.

Adequate Levels of Clotting Factors

A mixing study is done when there is a prolonged PT and/or PTT to determine if there is a coagulation factor inhibitor present. The patient sample is mixed in a 1:1 ratio with normal pooled plasma. If the test is corrected, a factor deficiency is present. If the test remains abnormal, an inhibitory substance is present.

Adequate Levels of Clotting Factors

Factor I

Factor I is also known as fibrinogen. Factor I deficiency is inherited in an autosomal recessive manner. Since Factor I is part of the common pathway, laboratory testing will indicate that both the PT and PTT will be prolonged.

Factor II (Prothrombin)

Factor II is also known as prothrombin. Factor II deficiency is inherited in an autosomal recessive manner. Since Factor II is part of the common pathway, laboratory testing will indicate that both the PT and PTT will be prolonged.

Adequate Levels of Clotting Factors

Factor III (Tissue Factor)

Factor III is also known as tissue factor. There is not a recognized bleeding disorder associated with tissue factor deficiency.

Adequate Levels of Clotting Factors

Factor IV (Calcium)

Factor IV is also known as calcium. There is not a recognized bleeding disorder associated with calcium deficiency.

Adequate Levels of Clotting Factors

Factor V

Factor V deficiency is also known as parahemophilia. Factor V deficiency is inherited in an autosomal recessive manner. Since factor V is part of the common pathway both the PT and PTT are typically prolonged. FFP is used for treatment. There is no Factor V concentrate.

Adequate Levels of Clotting Factors

Factor VI

Factor VI is the same as Factor Va and is also known as Accelerin. There is not a recognized bleeding disorder associated with factor VI deficiency.

Adequate Levels of Clotting Factors

Factor VII

Diagnosis: Factor VII deficiency is inherited in an autosomal recessive manner. Since Factor VII is part of the extrinsic pathway, the PT is typically prolonged but the PTT is normal. Factor VII deficiency is treated with recombinant factor VIIa concentrate.

Adequate Levels of Clotting Factors

Factor VIII

Factor VIII deficiency is also known as hemophilia. It is inherited in a X-linked recessive manner. Since factor VIII is part of the intrinsic pathway, the PTT will be pronged but the PT will be normal.

Factor IX

Factor IX deficiency is also known as hemophilia B. It is inherited in a X-linked recessive manner. Since factor IX is part of the intrinsic pathway, the PTT will be pronged but the PT will be normal.

Adequate Levels of Clotting Factors

Factor X

Factor X deficiency is inherited in an autosomal recessive manner. Factor X is part of the common pathway therefore both the PT and PTT are prolonged.

Factor XI

Factor XI deficiency is also known as Hemophilia C. It differs from hemophilia A or B in that there is no bleeding into joints and muscles. Factor XI deficiency is more common than hemophilia A and B in women and is therefore the second most common bleeding disorder affecting women after von Willebrand disease. It is inherited in a autosomal recessive manner. Since factor XI is part of the intrinsic clotting system, the PTT is prolonged and the PT is normal. There is factor XI recombinant protein available in Europe. In the US treatment consists of FFP.

Adequate Levels of Clotting Factors

Factor XII

Factor XII deficiency is not associated with any significant bleeding issues. It is inherited in an autosomal recessive manner. Since Factor XII is part of the intrinsic pathway, the PT is normal and the PTT is prolonged. These patients do not bleed excessively.

Factor XIII

Factor XIII deficiency is inherited in an autosomal recessive manner. In Factor XIII deficiency both the PT and PTT will be normal. The clot solubility will be abnormal. The clinical course of this disease is variable. It can be associated with abnormal bleeding in some patients. Factor XIII concentrate, FFP or cryoprecipitate for replacement therapy or for treatment of acute bleeding episodes.

Adequate Levels of Clotting Factors

Prekallekrein

Prekallikrein is a contact factor that complexes with high molecular weight kininogen and is cleaved by factor XII (Hageman factor) to produce kallikrein in the initial steps of the intrinsic pathway. Prekallekrien deficiency is inherited in an autosomal recessive fashion. These patients do not have any significant bleeding issues. This abnormality is associated with an prolonged PTT and a normal PT.

HMWK

High molecular weight kininogen is a protein produced by the liver that is involved in the early steps of the intrinsic coagulation pathway. HMWK functions as a cofactor and binds with prekallikrein and factor XI to help facilitate their activation by factor XIIa. These patients do not have any significant bleeding issues. This disorder is inherited in an autosomal recessive manner. Since HMWK is part of the instrisic pathway, the PTT will be prolonged and the PT will be normal. No treatment is necessary.

Adequate Levels of Clotting Factors

Von Willebrand Disease

Von Willebrand disease is characterized by
insufficient or ineffective von Willebrand
factor leading to impaired platelet adhesion
and deficient factor VIII levels. There are
different types of VWD that are characterized
by deficient or dysfunctional von Willebrand
factor. Since von Willebrand factor assists in
the stabilization of Factor VIII, this disorder is
associated with decreased factor VIII levels.
The disease is typically characterized by a
proloned PTT and a normal PT.

Factor II Inhibitor

Acquired prothrombin (Factor II) inhibitors are most commonly seen in in patients with antiphospholipid antibodies. They are often detected because of prolongation of the thrombin time. Prothrombin (Factor II) inhibitors can be associated with significant clinical bleeding although they are often detected incidentally in patients without clinical bleeding.

<u>Adequate Levels of Clotting Factors</u>

Factor V Inhibitor

Factor V inhibitors often develop after exposure to topical fibrin glues or bovine thrombin preparations that are contaminated with bovine factor. Other associated conditions included cancer, autoimmune disease, the postpartum state, and inherited factor V deficiency.

Adequate Levels of Clotting Factors

Thrombin Antibodies

Thrombin antibodies can develop after exposure to bovine thrombin found in topical thrombin or fibrin-glue preparations although they have been described in patients with other autoimmune disorders who have not had exposure to topical thrombin. These antibodies do not typically cause clinical bleeding although these they can cause severe bleeding. The thrombin time is prolonged when using bovine reagent thrombin. The PTT is prolonged and the prothrombin time will be increased if Factor V inhibitors are also present.

Factor VIII Inhibotrs

Factor VIII inhibitors are the most common autoantibodies that are associated with clinical bleeding. Spontaneous hemarthrosis are unusual. Common symptoms include hematomas and ecchymoses. Other symptoms include severe mucosal bleeding including epistaxis, gastrointestinal bleeding and gross hematuria.

Adequate Levels of Clotting Factors

Factor VIII Inhibitors

Factor VIII inhibitor treatment is composed of immunosuppression in an attempt to decreases the inhibitor titer. The most commonly used treatment protocols include steroids. Glucocorticoids can be used alone or with cyclophosphamide or rituximab.

Adequate Levels of Clotting Factors

Vitamin K Deficiency

Vitamin K deficiency is characterized by a deficiency of multiple vitamin K dependent factors, both procoagulant and anticoagulant. These vitamin K dependent factors include factor II, VII, IX, X, protein S, protein C. Since the vitamin dependent factors include components of the intrinsic, extrinsic, and common anticoagulation pathway, the PT and PTT are both prolonged.

DIC

Disseminated intravascular coagulation (DIC) is characterized by excessive generation of thrombin and fibrin with increased platelet aggregation and consumption of coagulation factors. When DIC develops over weeks or months is associated with venous thrombotic and embolic manifestations. When DIC develops over hours or days bleeding is more likely to develop.

Adequate Levels of Clotting Factors

DIC

Laboratory abnormalities include thrombocytopenia associated with a prolonged PT and PTT. Patients typically have elevated plasma d-dimer associated with a low plasma fibrinogen level. DIC is treated by addressing the underlying cause along with correction of the cause and replacement of platelets, coagulation factors (in fresh frozen plasma), and fibrinogen (in cryoprecipitate) to control severe bleeding.

<u>Adequate Levels of Clotting Factors</u>

Liver Failure

A coagulopathy can develop in liver failure
because the liver is involved in producing the
majority of the coagulation factors including
factors in the intrinsic, extrinsic and common
pathways. Because of this, both the PT and
the PTT are prolonged. The PT is more
sensitive in measuring liver failure and
coagulopathy because factor VII, produced by
the liver, is the coagulation factor with the
shortest half-life. For this reason, the PT is the
first test to abnormally prolonged.

Adequate Levels of Clotting Factors

Summary

The X-linked recessive factor deficiencies are Factor VIII and Factor IX deficiency.

Adequate Levels of Clotting Factors

Summary

The autosomal recessive factor deficiencies include Factor II, Factor V, Factor VII, Factor X, Factor XI, and Fibrinogen.

Adequate Levels of Clotting Factors

Summary

Additional autosomal recessive factor deficiencies include Factor XIII deficiency. This disorder is associated with bleeding and impaired wound healing. Patients with factor XIII deficiency will have a normal PT and a normal PTT, but an abnormal clot solubility.

Adequate Levels of Clotting Factors

Summary

Factor XII, prekallekrein, and HMWK are other autosomal recessive Factor deficiencies. These abnormalities are associated with prolonged PTT but are not associated with any excessive clinical bleeding.

Stages of Hemostasis

Vessel Wall Integrity

Adequate Numbers of Platelets

Proper Functioning Platelets

Adequate Levels of Clotting Factors

Proper Function of Fibrinolytic Pathway

Anticoagulation Effect

Fibrinolysis

Fibrinolysis is an important stage of the coagulation system that down-regulates coagulation. Fibrinolysis is mediated by tPA and urokinase. Fibrinolysis is regulated by plasminogen activator inhibitors (PAIs) and plasmin inhibitors like α2-antiplasmin. If fibrinolysis is not down regulated, bleeding can occur.

Reduced PAI-1 levels or reduced α2-antiplasmin can result in increased fibrinolysis characterized by a bleeding.

Alpha 2 Antiplasmin Deficiency

Alpha 2 Antiplasmin deficiency is an autosomal recessive disorder that can be associated with excessive bleeding. Plasminogen is activated by tissue-type plasminogen activator (tPA) and urokinase-type plasminogen activator (uPA). Plasminogen is converted into plasmin, which causes cleavage of insoluble fibrin polymers at specific sites, resulting in soluble fragments. The main physiological inhibitor of plasmin is alpha 2-antiplasmin and to some extent α2-macroglobulin. Alpha 2-antiplasmin is a natural inhibitor of plasmin in human circulation and plays a key role in the regulation of fibrinolysis.

Alpha 2 Antiplasmin Deficiency

The plasmin-antiplasmin system regulates the dissolution of fibrin polymers into soluble fragments. Patients with Alpha 2 antiplasmin deficiency will have a normal PT and PTT. The clot solubility will be abnormal. Alpha 2-antiplasmin deficiency is usually treated effectively with antifibrinolytic agents such as aminocaproic acid or tranexamic acid.

PAI-1 Deficiency

Plasminogen activator inhibitor-1 (PAI-1) deficiency . This is an autosomal recessive disorder. Plasminogen activators, urokinase plasminogen activator (u-PA) and tissue plasminogen activator (t-PA), circulate in plasma as a reversible complex with PAI-1. When the fibrin clot is formed, plasminogen and t-PA or u-PA bind to the clot and form plasmin which results in lysis of the cross linked fibrin to fibrin degradation products. PAI-1 also binds to fibrin and when bound, can irreversibly inhibit plasminogen activators.

<u>Proper Function of Fibrinolytic Pathway</u>

PAI-1 Deficiency

The PT and PTT are both normal. The clot solubility will be abnormal. PAI-1 deficiency can be safely and efficiently managed with antifibrinolytic therapy. Both epsilon-amino caproic acid (EACA) and tranexamic acid (TA) have been documented to control and prevent bleeding.

Stages of Hemostasis

Vessel Wall Integrity

Adequate Numbers of Platelets

Proper Functioning Platelets

Adequate Levels of Clotting Factors

Proper Function of Fibrinolytic Pathway

Anticoagulation Effect

Anticoagulation Effect

Dabigatran

Dabigatran (Pradaxa) is a direct thrombin inhibitor. The PT/INR and PTT will be prolonged in patients on this medication. Dabigatran has no effect on the anti-Xa assay. A commercial dilute Thrombin Time (Hemoclot) could possibly be used for monitoring. Dabigatran can be removed with dialysis in the setting of overdose.

Anticoagulation Effect

Rovaroxaban

Rivaroxaban (Xeralto) is a Factor Xa inhibitor. Rivaroxaban will prolong the PT and PTT. The modified anti-Xa assay is required for use in Rivaroxaban testing.

Anticoagulation Effect

Apixiban

Apixaban (Eliquis) is a Factor Xa inhibitor. This medication prolongs the PT and PTT. Factor Xa chromogenic assays show high sensitivity and a linear correlation.

Anticoagulation Effect

Edoxaban

Edoxaban (Savaysa) is a factor Xa inhibitor. Edoxaban prolongs the PT and PTT. Anti-Xa activity is used for edoxaban quantification.

This concludes Diagnosis of the Bleeding
Patient: Fast Focus Study Guide

Search Amazon Kindle books to find other
study guides written by
JT Thomas, MD

Internal Medicine Study Guide
Hematology Study Guide
Medical Oncology Study Guide
Cardiology Study Guide
Multiple Myeloma Study Guide
Differential Diagnosis Study Guide
Rheumatology Study Guide
Cancer Study Guide

www.ingramcontent.com/pod-product-compliance
Lightning Source LLC
Chambersburg PA
CBHW070829180526
45168CB00002B/785